Coping with Stress

D1799556

CANCELLED

Dr G Wilkinson

This is a Family Doctor booklet published by the British Medical Association, BMA House, Tavistock Square, London WC1H 9JR

ISBN: 0 7279 0138 9

Typeset and printed in Great Britain by
Latimer Trend & Company Ltd, Plymouth

Contents

Coping with stress	5
Levels of stress	7
Sources of stress	9
Recognising the warning signs	15
Tackling the problem	19
Defences against stress	21
Social support	29
False friends	37
Conclusion	46

Editor: Norma Pearce
Medical Editor: Dr Tony Smith
Design: Lloyd Fishwick Associates

Life events and stress*

Events	Stress rating
Death of spouse Divorce Marital separation Jail term Death of close family member Personal injury or illness Marriage Loss of job	Highest
Marital reconciliation Retirement Change in health of family member Pregnancy Sex difficulties Gain of new family member Business readjustment Change of financial state Death of close friend	High
Change in number of arguments with spouse Mortgage of over £20 000 Foreclosure of mortgage or loan Change in responsibilities at work Son or daughter leaving home Trouble with in-laws Outstanding personal achievement Wife begins or stops work Begin or end of school Change in living conditions Revision of personal habits Trouble with boss	Moderate
Change in work hours or conditions Change of residence Change in schools Change in recreation Change in church activities Change in social activities Mortgage or loan less than £20 000 Change in sleeping habits Change in number of family gatherings Change in eating habits Vacation Christmas	Low
Minor violations of the law	Lowest

*Holmes and Rahe

Coping with stress

What is stress? Anything that makes you tense, angry, frustrated, or miserable. It may be the prospect of a driving test or a visit from a difficult relative; the uncertainties and decisions inevitable in moving house or getting married; or the unavoidable burdens of coping with a death in the family. Factors that stress some people give others excitement; racing drivers and mountaineers seem to thrive on physical challenges, while some businessmen get thrills from takeover battles or devising new advertising campaigns. One man's stress may be another man's pleasure.

A certain amount of stress is desirable to give us the required stimulation and motivation to overcome the many obstacles that may prevent us achieving our goals, and to alleviate boredom—we often deliberately create mild stress in our lives to help overcome periods of frustration and dull routine.

Too much stress, however, affects our health and wellbeing, everyday performance, and outward social behaviour adversely. Over time we may be weakened by recurrent, prolonged, or severe stress and because of this find it more difficult to adapt to change.

How we respond to pressure is determined by our

characters; by our personal disabilities or illnesses. These dictate how we react to difficulties with relationships, both at home and at work, and to practical problems over money, work, and housing.

Overcoming stress

The principal remedies used to reduce and overcome stress are straightforward, and in most cases self-help methods are very successful. Although almost everyone is under some form of stress, only a few ever respond by developing a physical or emotional illness that requires specialist help. There is every reason to be optimistic that you will be able to overcome the stress in your life.

A question of adjustment

As we grow and mature we learn ways of predicting and controlling most aspects of our everyday life. When unfamiliar circumstances arise we make adjustments in attitude and behaviour in order to understand and cope with them successfully. Usually this is fairly straightforward and we are hardly aware of the process. When events of major importance take place, however, such as marriage, birth, or the death of someone close, adjustment and adaptation are both more difficult and more obvious to us.

In order to live successfully with stress we should spend some time considering the sources of stress in our lives and whether our physical and psychological responses to these are appropriate and useful or are preventing us from coping and taking control. Although studies show that the ability to cope is largely inborn, it is also a question of training, environment, and practice.

Levels of stress

I have already stated that stress can be both a good thing—a motivator—and a bad thing. Furthermore, what is stressful may not only vary from one person to another but can change for one individual from year to year. This is because the way that stress is experienced depends on a balance between the demand made by the event causing the stress and the person's ability to cope (which can vary considerably). Too large an imbalance between demand and ability to cope may result in the sort of stress that is not good for us.

Stress equation
Looked at in a slightly different way, the overall level of stress is determined by a complicated equation that takes account of the stressful event (stressor), our response to this in terms of physical effects, emotions, and outward behaviour (stress response), and how significant the event is to us (is it something that makes us very happy, deeply sad, or is it not too important).

Level of stress = Environmental stressor	+ Stress response	+ Significance of event

For example if John Smith with a large mortgage, a wife and three children, and a job which he enjoys and is important to him is made redundant the level of stress he experiences may be high. The event is of major significance to him and he may suffer physical symptoms (inability to sleep, eat, or relax) and emotional reactions (frustration, aggression) which affect his outward behaviour. Jim Brown on the other hand,

Stress curve

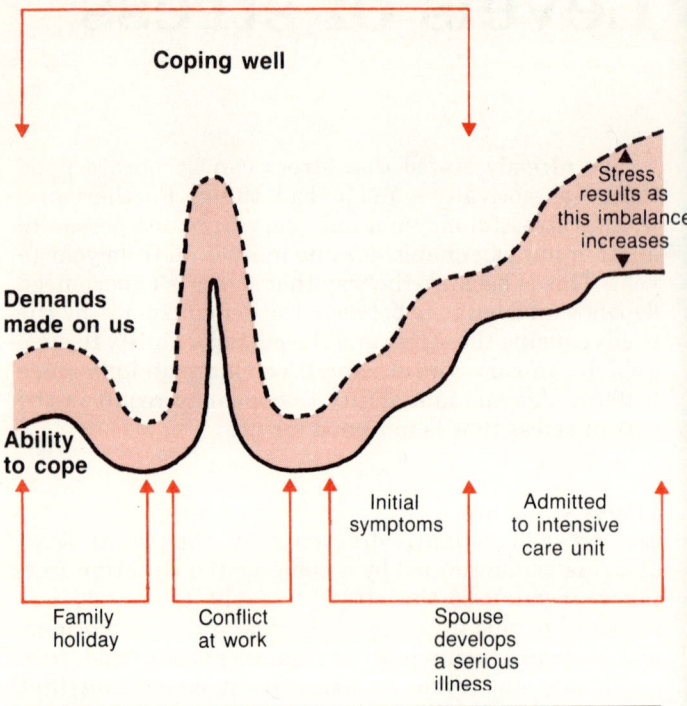

Too large an imbalance between the demands made on us and our ability to cope may result in the sort of stress that is not good for us.

is 23 with no responsibilities and a job which he finds boring. If he is made redundant, he may not be shattered. He may feel that the event has forced him to make a long overdue change and he may be relieved and cheerful and feel better than he has done in ages. In his case stress has a positive side and is needed to introduce a necessary element of change in his life. We can see from this that similar stressors may evoke an entirely different response in different people.

Sources of stress

We would all become extremely bored if nothing ever happened in our lives but too much change too quickly can be a major cause of stress—the demands outweigh our ability to cope. An indication of how much stress various typical life events and social changes may cause is given in the Table. In general the greater number we experience in a given time span such as a year and the higher their combined rating, the more likely we are to suffer a stress response, either physical or emotional. Moreover the severity of the stress response is usually related to the number and significance of the events and changes experienced. Remember that stress can be triggered off by events that are traditionally viewed as pleasant like getting married, winning money, or having a baby as well as by adverse events like losing a job or the illness of someone in the family.

Evaluating the impact of life events
When evaluating the impact of life events and social changes as a cause of stress we also need to take into account the fact that they tend to be particularly

Life events and stress*

Events	Stress rating
Death of spouse Divorce Marital separation Jail term Death of close family member Personal injury or illness Marriage Loss of job	**Highest**
Marital reconciliation Retirement Change in health of family member Pregnancy Sex difficulties Gain of new family member Business readjustment Change of financial state Death of close friend	**High**
Change in number of arguments with spouse Mortgage of over £20 000 Foreclosure of mortgage or loan Change in responsibilities at work Son or daughter leaving home Trouble with in-laws Outstanding personal achievement Wife begins or stops work Begin or end of school Change in living conditions Revision of personal habits Trouble with boss	**Moderate**
Change in work hours or conditions Change of residence Change in schools Change in recreation Change in church activities Change in social activities Mortgage or loan less than £20 000 Change in sleeping habits Change in number of family gatherings Change in eating habits Vacation Christmas	**Low**
Minor violations of the law	**Lowest**

*Holmes and Rahe

stressful when they are:

Unpredictable   **Unfamiliar**
Of great magnitude   **Of great intensity**
We feel impelled to undergo or be subjected to them

Do be careful, however, not to take the contents of the Table too literally. It is common for people who feel stressed to search for the reason in past events but these may be the result rather than the cause of the stress. The feeling of not being able to cope with new duties or responsibilities, for example, may be the result of unrecognised depression rather than the depression being the result of a failure to cope.

The sources of stress, therefore, lie mainly in these environmental stressors and in our physical and psychological responses to them. The cause may be obvious to us, in which case the process of adaptation may be straightforward and clear cut and depend on making practical or emotional adjustments. Furthermore, in these circumstances it may be easy to see where help should be sought from.

Often, though, the source lies hidden from our immediate view and it may require some careful thought or discussion with others to bring it to the surface. Again, unrecognised depression may reduce the ability to cope or there may be difficulties with relationships that we are not prepared to face. Sometimes we may never find an answer—very occasionally stress does come "out of the blue".

Find the factors affecting you

Begin by sitting down and asking yourself whether there are any environmental, social, physical, or emotional factors that are affecting you.

- How much are you smoking?
- How much alcohol are you drinking?
- How little exercise are you taking?

- Could you be ill?
- Is there some new element in your life?
- Has there been any change in your general circumstances?
- Have long standing problems recently become more acute?
- Is someone close to you facing difficulties that affect you?

Life phases
You may get a clue from considering the phase of life you are in—in adolescence many major decisions have to be made for the first time; in midlife responsibilities are often heaviest and most dramatic; and in old age there may be illness, bereavement, and poverty to cope with alone. You should also consider the phases of life that those close to you are in.

Conflicts
Ask yourself whether you have any important conflicts that you need to resolve: do you have conflicting views or opinions about someone or something? Is some situation leaving you with a feeling of personal inadequacy or guilt? Are you taking or being made to take a new or unaccustomed role—or perhaps you are carrying or being asked to carry too much responsibility. Do you have unexpressed fears or frustrations about your life?

Often stress is the result of an accumulation of related and unrelated factors of these kinds. If you settle down quietly and list the stresses in your life you may be surprised—and relieved—by discovering that some of the stresses are ones that you can eliminate.

Mental defence mechanisms

Adaptation is a two-stage process. Firstly we have to realise that some of our repeated responses to continuing stress may be unhelpful: secondly, we need to explore and use new ways of coping until satisfactory solutions are found.

Some of these unhelpful, repeated responses—*defence mechanisms*—are described below. Remember though, that these are merely concepts that may help us understand ourselves by giving insight into the way our minds work and how we react to stress.

Compensation—the development of a personal quality to offset a defect or sense of inferiority. Overcompensation occurs when compensation is overdone. An excessively conscientious and scrupulous person, for example, may be compensating for contrary tendencies.

Conversion—the manifestation of hidden fears in the form of bodily symptoms. Someone who is afraid of going out may develop a weakness in the legs.

Denial—persuading oneself that there is nothing amiss when, in fact, there is, in the hope that the trouble will somehow be removed or simply go away (out of sight, out of mind).

Displacement—the shifting of emotion from one target to another. Ideas or attitudes which make us uncomfortable may be disguised or avoided in this way. For example, anger with our workmates may be taken out on our spouse or family.

Dissociation—we avoid looking too closely at attitudes so that inconsistencies in our thought and conduct are overlooked.

Fixation—personal characteristics are fixed at levels appropriate to earlier, less mature periods. In this way childish methods of reacting to difficulties, excessive dependence on others, and self-centred behaviour may be retained in later life.

Identification—conscious or unconscious modelling of oneself on another person, which may include the assumption of his or her dress, leisure activities, etc. This may be quite normal; for example, young people often imitate the attitudes and behaviour of older persons whom they regard highly.

Introjection—turning inwards of feelings and attitudes towards others which give rise to conflict and aggression. Hostility towards others may then take the form of self harm or self destructiveness.

Inversion—the exaggeration of tendencies opposite to those which are repressed (see below). Prudery, for example, may be an inversion of repressed sexual desire.

Projection—the opposite of introjection, the displacement of personal attitudes on to others or the environment. This is another way of avoiding self blame and guilty feelings. Personal inadequacies are blamed on others or the environment.

Rationalisation—a form of self deception in which socially acceptable reasons are found for conduct prompted by less worthy motives.

Regression—a reversion to ways of thinking, feeling, and behaving which are more appropriate to earlier stages of individual or social development. Thus, an adult may regress to childish temper tantrums.

Repression—the thrusting out of consciousness of ideas and impulses which are incompatible with what the individual regards as correct in the circumstances. Repression is unconscious and involuntary, in contrast to *suppression*, which is a willed checking or inhibition of thoughts, feelings, and actions which conflict with moral standards.

Resistance—the barrier between the unconscious and the conscious mind, preventing resolution of incompatible mental elements. For example, someone might unconsciously resist enquiring into the origins of his stress, thereby prolonging his condition.

Sublimation—the direction of undesirable or forbidden tendencies into more socially acceptable channels. For example, childish self-indulgent behaviour is sublimated into altruistic social behaviour in the process of maturity. Surplus energy may be sublimated into useful channels.

Transferance—the experience of emotions towards one person which are derived from experience with another. For example, anxious or hostile feelings previously felt towards a domineering parent may in later life be felt in relation to authority figures.

Withdrawal—giving up, and physical and emotional retirement from a stressful situation, characterised by loss of enthusiasm and interest, apathy, and day dreaming.

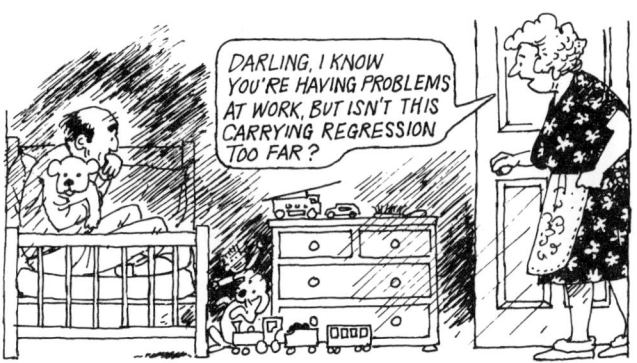

Recognising the warning signs of stress

The warning signs that stress may be affecting your health vary considerably from person to person. Most of us, however, have a quite well defined personal stress response or "finger print"—maybe headaches, or an outbreak of eczema, or diarrhoea. Usually the first signs of stress are changes in our emotional life or behaviour. Our personal characteristics, attitudes, and peculiarities may become more noticeable (often to others rather than ourselves).

Emotional reactions

The most important changes to watch out for are increases in tension, irritability, and moodiness. Small irritations may seem unbearable if they come on top of stress and can cause a major outburst or upset. The fact that the children want to play Monopoly when you have just come home from work, for example, seems to merit putting them up for adoption; you have an overwhelming desire to perpetrate grievous bodily harm on your car when it refuses to start; and when the toaster will not eject your slice of toast you have to be restrained from attacking it with the bread knife.

There may also be changes in appetite and therefore weight: some people lose interest in food whereas others have a constant desire to eat. Effectiveness and ability to cope at home and at work may become extremely variable: you can't quite get round to paying the household bills and are spurred into action only when the phone is disconnected; and the brain seems to have moved into reverse gear at work so that the "in tray" gets bigger and bigger. You smoke or drink (or both) more, which does, however, help fill in the time in the evening as you seem to have difficulty in sleeping.

If you notice some of these signs of stress, or other people point them out to you, take heed; unless you take steps to protect yourself you are at risk of experiencing increasing stress. You may not recognise all the signs at first, however, or you may have overlooked or ignored some for a variety of reasons. Moreover, you may also have to resist a tendency to regard the reactions as definite evidence of serious physical illness rather than a response to stress. The Table lists possible emotional and intellectual reactions to stress.

Emotional and intellectual reactions to stress

Subjective awareness of being under pressure
Feeling tense or under threat and unable to relax
Feeling mentally drained
Constantly frightened or terrified
Increasing irritability and complaining
Feeling of conflict
Frustration and aggression
Restlessness, increasing inability to concentrate or
    complete tasks quickly
Increased tearfulness
Becoming more fussy, pessimistic, gloomy, or suspicious
Increasing indecision
Impulses to run and hide
Fears of imminent fainting, collapse, or death
Fears of social embarrassment or failure
Lack of ability to feel pleasure or enjoyment

Physical reactions

Physical reactions to strong emotions were designed to
save us in the days when we led the simple, dangerous
life of the caveman. To prehistoric man these bodily
responses meant "fight or flight" and prepared him for
action; millions of years later they still do—very useful
if a dinosaur is on the rampage but not a great deal of
help when we have just missed the last train or dropped
the car keys down a drain in the road. What happens is
that our pulse and blood pressure increase, we breathe
more rapidly, and our sensory organs (ears, eyes, nose)
become more alert. These changes are thought to be
controlled by the action of stress hormones released
into the blood circulation in response to the stressful
stimuli.

When this stress response is prolonged or occurs
frequently and under inappropriate circumstances a
wide range of unpleasant feelings can ensue. The
number and nature of the feelings differ greatly

between people but the most common are set out in the Table.

Physical reactions to stress

Change in appetite	Nausea and squeamishness
Sleep difficulties	Startling
Headaches	Weakness of the limbs
Indigestion	Frequent urge to pass urine
Rapid, erratic, or more pronounced heart beat	Muscle weakness or trembling
Chest discomfort	Muscle tension
Constipation or diarrhoea	Odd aches, pains, or twitches
Worsening of long standing discomforts or pain	Tiredness and weakness
	Sweating
Backache	Constant restlessness and fidgeting
Breathlessness	
"Butterflies" in the stomach	"Pins and needles" in hands or feet
Dry mouth or throat	

Social and behavioural reactions to stress

The social behaviour of people under stress can change quite considerably. Often they hate to be alone and make efforts to seek out support from family and friends, or, in contrast, may become withdrawn and indifferent. They seem to have lost interest in others and begin to refuse invitations because they are too much trouble.

People under stress can become indecisive (a trip to the supermarket for a packet of tea bags seems to require as much thought and preparation as the ascent of Everest) and continually seeking reassurance. They can be capricious (they may speak fondly of someone one moment and find them completely unworthy the next). They may be tearful, difficult, and complaining and often expect others to be impossibly understanding. The fairly "relaxed" person may become rigid and obsessive, indulging in excessive checking of locks and switches, for example, or cleaning the oven at three in the morning when previously it was done once a year.

This may be in an effort to bring some order and certainty to the atmosphere of confusion which they feel is predominating.

There may be a change in sexual habits (a loss of interest, increase in casual sex, or altered sexual preference) and the previously mild mannered may become verbally or physically aggressive.

Often the person under stress denies these behavioural changes but they are usually very obvious to others. Ask a friend if they have noticed any of these facets in your behaviour, but don't be cross with them for telling the truth—remember that denying the obvious is a sign of stress!

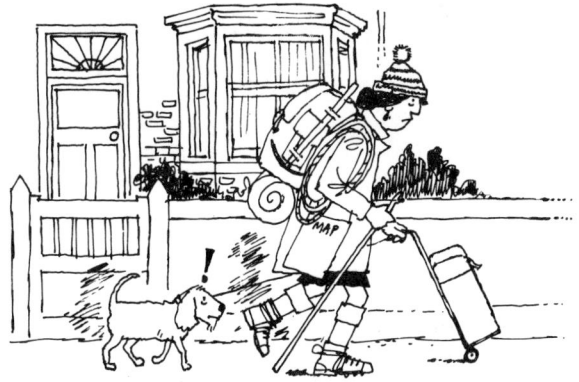

"A trip to the supermarket for a packet of tea bags seems to require as much thought and preparation as the ascent of Everest"

Tackling the problem

The most difficult thing about stress is recognising it: doing something about it is relatively easy. Once you have recognised that you are suffering a stress response identify and tackle the underlying causes, not just the symptoms. It may be helpful to have the opinion of someone you can trust and respect in this activity.

Make a list

First of all list all your signs of stress, noting how severe they are and how long they have lasted for. Next list all the possible causes and sort them into categories. Is the cause a *major life event*, for example bereavement? Is there a serious *problem* such as redundancy or what to do about elderly parents who can no longer look after themselves? Are you troubled by a *worry* such as a teenage daughter who has abandoned her A level physics and maths course and gone to London to become a model? Or have you been beleaguered by a series of *irritations*—they have been drilling the street for three weeks, you are having difficulty keeping up at work because you have a new colleague who needs help, the children refuse to do their homework before you have spent 10 minutes nagging them each night and even then you have to check it. Remember that a series of minor irritations may be more disorientating than the major problems of life.

Having categorised all the possible causes of your stress you can sort them into those that have a practical solution, those that will resolve themselves given time, and those that you can do nothing to change. You should try to let go of those that fall into the second and third groups—what you cannot change try to stop worrying about; your teenage daughter may give up her attempts to be a model and go back to college or she may be so successful she becomes a millionairess, and the drilling outside may be a distant memory a month from now. Where there are practical solutions (and this applies to most *problems*) make a list of these and try them out.

You should be prepared for the fact that *some of these solutions may upset others*. Remember that looking after yourself does not mean being unkind to others and that you are only useful to yourself and to others if you are functioning well.

Monitor progress

The next stage is to monitor your stress response by keeping a note of the changes in the nature, severity, or duration of the signs. After a week repeat the process to see how you are getting on: if some of the solutions do not seem to be working try alternative ones. Keep assessing progress until you feel that you have reduced as many of the causes of stress as possible and that you are in control of things.

Defences against stress

We can defend ourselves against stress in our lives by understanding what causes us stress and by learning how to avoid or adjust and adapt better to this. The principle defences are within ourselves and mainly consist of physical and mental fitness—a healthy body and a healthy mind.

Physical defences

We can improve our defences by leading a healthy, enjoyable life, and looking after ourselves.

Sleep

Firstly, we should ensure that we get enough sleep and should learn how to relax (see page 26). Sleep does knit up the ravelled sleeve of care. The amount needed varies from person to person, but it is probably true to say that more is needed during times of stress than when life is running quietly and smoothly—beware, however, of taking too much sleep, it can make you feel almost as bad as too little. Sleeping problems are very common among those under stress but do make sure that you do not worry unnecessarily about a few bad nights—you can usually catch up after one good night's sleep.

If you are having difficulty in sleeping make sure that you eat supper early and avoid strong tea or coffee (unless it is decaffeinated) after 7 pm. Try to tire yourself physically, have a bath, and then spend some time switching your mind off before going to bed by reading or watching television, or even playing patience. Do not allow yourself to brood over problems, they can wait until the morning! If you can't get to sleep or wake in the middle of the night and can't get to sleep again, get up, make yourself a drink (preferably not tea or coffee), have another game of patience or do some mindless chore like cleaning the oven or tidying the tool box and then go back to bed. Do not lie in bed worrying.

Try not to succumb to taking sleeping pills unless its only for one or two nights in order to break the pattern of sleeplessness. They may make you feel fuzzy and dopey in the morning and can develop into a dangerous habit!

Diet
We should eat a sensible diet to avoid the health hazards of being overweight and to reduce or prevent the risks of developing diseases known to be related to diet, such as heart disease, high blood pressure, bowel cancer, and late onset diabetes.

The main principles are to eat far less fat and fatty foods, especially those containing saturated fats and cholesterols; increase dietary fibre by eating more whole grain cereals, pulses and fresh fruit and vegetables; and cut down on sugar and salt. This can be

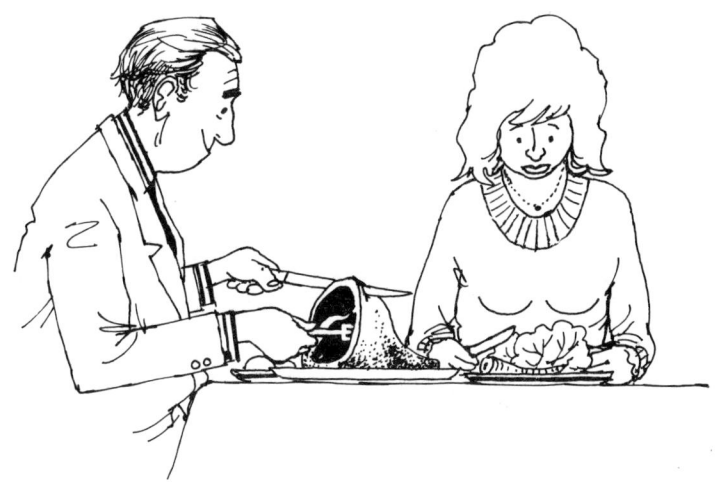

difficult as it goes against all that many of us hold dear such as the traditional Sunday lunch of roast beef, Yorkshire pudding, and roast potatoes! Don't go too quickly in your campaign for diet reform, change a few products at a time and add new foods rather than just cutting out those that you currently eat and are bad for you. If you live for Sunday roast lunch don't abandon it completely, changing your diet should not be a torture it should be fun!

Be careful about what you drink. Too much tea or coffee can be overstimulating, and excessive alcohol is certainly no friend to good health.

Exercise
There is only one way to keep the body trim and fit—by exercise. We all need some regular exercise, preferably daily. This might amount to no more than a pleasant, brisk 15 minute walk in the fresh air, but it could well be much more. At the very least you will be more likely to feel physically and mentally relaxed, to get a refreshing sleep, and your appetite will be stimulated. The important thing is that the exercise chosen should be pleasurable—which for some of us is a problem!

Whatever you decide to do in the way of exercise always bear the following points in mind:

1. Warm up for two or three minutes before starting by stretching or running on the spot;
2. Build up slowly and do not overextend yourself— always exercise within the limits of comfort (let your breathing be your guide);
3. If you feel excessively tired stop and rest, there is always tomorrow;
4. When stopping exercise cool down gradually and slowly to avoid stiffness;
5. Exercise sessions three times a week for about 20 minutes, at a pace that keeps you moderately "puffed" (not gasping for breath) are likely to be best for stimulating the muscles and circulation.

Mental defences

Improving general health and fitness can protect against and lessen the effects of stress. Some events are inherently stressful but many of our reactions to these depend on our attitudes, beliefs, and values. We have already considered defence mechanisms and how although these may be helpful in the short term, they may be a bar to adaptation and coping. Another approach to overcoming stress is to assume that we have difficulty in coping with change because we do not have appropriate or enough coping strategies available. We need to learn new skills of self instruction and self control.

Self instruction
When we learn a new skill, such as driving a car, we learn from a combination of receiving instruction and observation. At the beginning, we are usually instructed by someone else; then we repeat the process giving the instructions to ourselves; and, finally, we complete the activity "automatically" without consciously thinking of the instructions.

We can apply a similar process of observation—instruction—self instruction—automatic ability to our everyday thinking. For example, suppose we feel stressed about taking examinations or having job interviews.

First, using a little imagination before the event, we can pay attention to the way our thoughts tend to work when the stress is imminent. What are the things that we say to ourselves? Perhaps, "Oh, my God, what can I say?; I wish this was all over; I wish I hadn't started this; Two hours still to go; They must think I'm an idiot" etc.

Next, we can make a list or a note of positive, practical instructions that would be more useful. Such as, "I had better start writing" rather than "I'm very nervous"; or "These are my good points and these are things I want to emphasise" rather than "I don't know what they're looking for".

Thirdly, during the event, we instruct ourselves positively with the most useful instructions we have thought of beforehand instead of wasting time and energy panicking or ruminating on irrelevant thoughts. In time this process becomes "automatic".

Control

Having a sense of control over events lessens their stressful impact. True, there are some things over which we have no control but there is usually some aspect of a problem that we can change to our advantage, thereby reducing stressful feelings of helplessness.

Self control methods can be useful when we wish to alter particular aspects of our behaviour or response to people or events.

First, carefully observe the behaviour in question, for example always getting angry with Bloggins at work; or being irritable with the family at breakfast time; or regularly missing the train because you leave home with too little time to spare. Chart the circumstances in a diary made up for the purpose.

Now, think of practical ways in which you can

modify the behaviour. For example, take a deep breath and ask Bloggins if you can help him; make a point of saying something nice at breakfast; make sure you leave home in plenty of time to catch the train.

The next part of the process of self control involves reward. Choose something pleasant to reward yourself with when you change the behaviour in question and reach a certain predetermined standard—buy yourself a treat if you manage to catch your train every morning for a week!

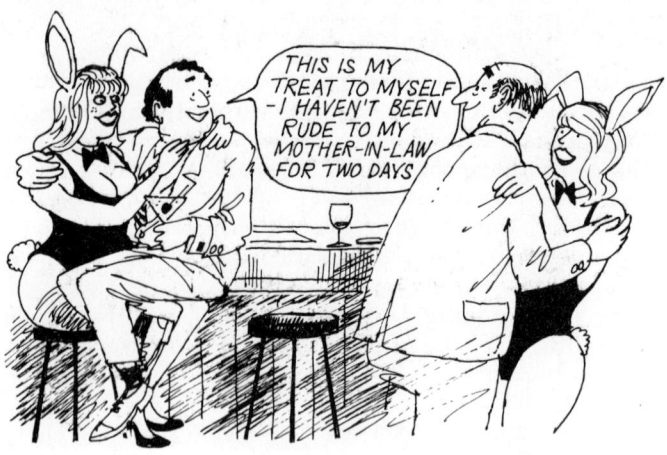

Relaxation

Relaxation is a most useful technique to practise when you feel under stress. There are a number of similar methods but one of the most widely used is described below. Read the instructions and familiarise yourself with them before having a go.

Do be patient and give yourself several tries before expecting the full beneficial results—for those of us who are very "twitchy" it can take time to learn how to relax.

Preparation

Sit in a comfortable chair or (even better) lie down somewhere comfortable in a quiet, warm room where you will not be interrupted.

If you are sitting, take off your shoes, uncross your legs, and rest your arms on the arms of the chair.

If you are lying down, lie on your back with your arms at your sides. If necessary use a comfortable pillow for your head.

Close your eyes and be aware of your body. Notice how you are breathing and where the muscular tensions are. Make sure you are comfortable.

Breathing

Start to breathe slowly and deeply, expanding your abdomen as you breathe *in*, then raising your rib cage to let more air in, till your lungs are filled right to the top. Hold your breath for a couple of seconds and then breathe *out* slowly, allowing your rib cage and stomach to relax, and empty your lungs completely.

Do not strain, with practise it will become much easier.

Keep this *slow, deep, rhythmic* breathing going throughout your relaxation session.

Relaxing

After five to 10 minutes, when you have your breathing pattern established, start the following sequence *tensing* each part of the body on an *in* breath, holding your breath for 10 seconds while you keep your muscles tense; then *relaxing* and breathing *out* at the same time.

1. Curl your toes hard and press your feet down

2. Press your heels down and bend your feet up

3. Tense your calf muscles

4. Tense your thigh muscles, straightening your knees and making your legs stiff

5. Make your buttocks tight

6. Tense your stomach as if to receive a punch

7. Bend your elbows and tense the muscles of your arms

8. Hunch your shoulders and press your head back into the cushion or pillow

9. Clench your jaws, frown, and screw up your eyes really tight

10. Tense all your muscles together

Remember to breathe deeply, and be aware when you relax of the feeling of physical wellbeing and heaviness spreading through your body.

After you have done the whole sequence (1–10) and still breathing slowly and deeply, imagine a white rose on a black background.

Try to "see" the rose as clearly as possible, concentrating your attention on it for 30 seconds. Do not hold your breath during this time, continue to breathe as you have been doing.

After this, go on to visualise a favourite, peaceful object of your choice in a similar fashion.

Lastly, give yourself the instruction that when you open your eyes you will be perfectly relaxed but alert.

Short routine
When you have become familiar with this technique, if you want to relax at any time when you have only a few minutes, do the sequence in shortened form, leaving out some muscle groups, but always working from your feet upwards. For example, you might do numbers 1, 4, 6, 8, and 10 if you do not have time to do the whole sequence.

Social support

Coping with stress can be made easier by having social support or help from family and friends—in fact the absence of this can itself create or contribute to stress. For example, feelings of uncertainty or anxiety about a particular situation can be increased by a belief that we are alone in the predicament; that there is no place or time to escape from the pressures; that no one else is interested; that no one else understands, or has faced and overcome similar difficulties; that having difficulty in coping with the situation is a sign of weakness and something to be ashamed of and hidden.

Social support can be found simply in having a stable home life, a trouble free environment at work, or some other "refuge" that provides a breathing space within which we can work through and resolve a particular stressful problem ourselves. Friendly or loving relationships can all bring the enjoyment and relaxation that help to counteract stress.

Having someone respected to talk to who will listen sympathetically and in confidence and who will, if required, provide moral support, practical advice, company, or simply distraction can be an enormous help in seeing a problem more clearly, in getting things in proportion, in exploring all possible solutions, and facing and getting through or learning to cope with stressful situations.

Loneliness
Of course, finding and benefiting from friendship and social support is not always easy. Loneliness and isolation may be difficult to break out of as fear of rejection can be deeply inhibiting. The important thing is to recognise the need for outside help, not to see this as a failure and something to be ashamed of.

If a well developed family and social network exists then we can learn how to use what it can provide to cope with stress. If an inherent part of the problem is one of isolation, then a network of social support can be developed by offering friendship and support to others and receiving it from them in return, by pursuing hobbies and interests which involve contact with other people of similar tastes, and by seeking intellectual and physical stimulation through classes, courses, sports, voluntary work, or political activities.

None of these steps are easy and all involve making a conscious effort to look outward, to be open and receptive to others, and optimistic and resilient in the face of difficulties, but they can in time be extremely beneficial and rewarding. Try not to forget that there are other people just as isolated and with just as much potential for giving as ourselves: to find them we must come out of ourselves.

Caring agencies
If as well as loneliness and isolation some more serious or specific difficulty is involved, then the various caring agencies can also provide support on a temporary or more long-term basis, for example your doctor, the churches, the Salvation Army, Social Services departments, citizen's advice bureaux, the Samaritans, and marriage guidance councils. There are, in addition, a number of national organisations that offer help, advice, and information about particular conditions or problems and they will usually be able to give you further details about local facilities. Your library

should have a copy of the Mental Health Foundation's *Someone to Talk to Directory*, 1985, which lists all these groups, or the College of Health (01 980 4848) can provide similar information. The essential thing is to try to identify the source of stress in your life, decide what kind of help you think would be best for you, and seek help from the people or agencies that you feel most comfortable about approaching. Also, try to recognise that like you, the people you turn to will have different strengths and weaknesses, and if you feel that a particular approach is not working say so to see if it can be changed or (preferably by mutual agreement) try elsewhere. Do not be deterred if your first approach does not bring an "instant" solution—keep trying.

Counselling

Counselling is a process covering a range of activities in which an attempt is made to understand the meaning of some event or state of being to an individual, family, or group and to plan, with the person or people concerned, how to manage the emotional and practical realities which face them. The purpose is not to impose a lifestyle but to assist the person to live the life he or she has consciously chosen. In practice, counselling and social support are inextricably linked.

Since almost anyone can set themselves up as a counsellor it is wise to ensure beforehand that the person you choose is trained, qualified, and experienced. You can do this by asking for advice from your doctor, minister of religion, or one of the self help agencies.

There are many different counselling techniques but the main characteristics of a successful counsellor are emotional warmth, understanding, and genuineness.

Reassurance
This is still probably the most widely used form of counselling. Bland reassurance is seldom if ever useful but careful listening will help identify the main stress

and then reassurance can consist of giving "new" information which is relevant to reducing the stress, put in a form which is easy to understand and remember.

Behavioural counselling
Behavioural counselling aims to change behaviour that is regarded as unacceptable. The main concern is to relieve a specific difficulty or symptom by studying the patterns of behaviour that led to difficulty and then modifying responses by learning more useful ways of dealing with problems. The accent is on doing rather than "just talking".

People with difficulty or inadequacy in their personal relationships (for example, shyness or embarrassment) can learn useful new "social skills" in this way. After discussing and observing your behaviour, the therapist may first explain the effects of this on other people, perhaps using a videotape of you to show you how you function. When you have together identified the problems in your approach, the therapist may then coach you in new more effective ways of behaving, and get you to act them out in a "role play" with others. Alternatively, the therapist may ask you to take on the role of someone who you have particular difficulties with, in an effort to help you to see more clearly and from a different angle how your own responses work.

Humanistic counselling
This is concerned with "personal growth" and helping us to achieve our full potential. Workers in this form of counselling make use of encounter groups, and personal therapy, massage, meditation, dancing, co-counselling, and virtually any method which seems likely to help people under stress to understand themselves more clearly and to feel better. The main aim is to integrate the health and wellbeing of the person as a whole.

Rational-emotive counselling
Rational-emotive counselling considers the way in

which we "worry about being worried". It involves identifying the irrational ways in which we think about problems and then helps us find less stress-provoking ways of dealing with our problems.

Rogerian counselling
This is not based on telling us what to do but on helping us work out for ourselves what we want and how best to achieve it. The counsellor's job is to facilitate self-understanding by "mirroring-back" to us our own understanding, to help us to reshape our thoughts and feelings, to share our experiences, and to discuss their development with us.

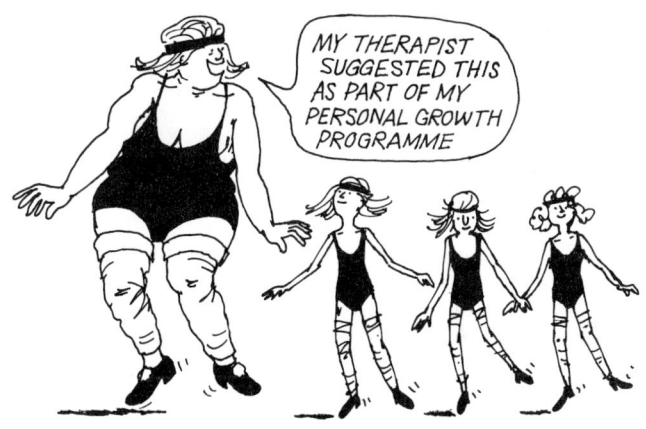

Self help groups

These are groups of people who feel they have a problem in common and have joined together to do something about it. They are small, voluntary groups for mutual aid and the accomplishment of some aim, and provide members with the following help.

Emotional support
People with stressful problems can feel lonely, con-
fused, and isolated and it helps to talk about these
problems with others "in the same boat". Support may
be given individually or communally. It may be aimed
at helping the individual to adjust to a situation or to
take steps to change it. It may be offered in crises or
may be available over a longer term.

Information and advice
For most of the problems with which self help groups
are concerned, there is a wealth of information to help
people cope more easily.

Direct services
Some forms of help needed to cope with particular
problems can be provided directly by mutual aid organisations. These may be provided on a casual or infor-
mal basis (for example baby sitting) or they may be
provided more formally (established playgroups). They
may be carried out by group members on a voluntary
basis or they may involve hired staff. A few groups even
provide services jointly with their local authority.

Pressure group activities
Many self help groups consider that the benefits and
services provided by the state are inadequate and form
a pressure group to bring about favourable changes.

Religious organisations

For many people under stress there is a natural tendency to turn to religion for solace and support. For
those who believe, the strength of shared belief and the
sense of belonging and common purpose can overcome
adversity and demoralisation.

Ministers of religion usually have great experience in counselling for a wide range of life's difficulties, and are often more than willing to talk things over with members of their flock.

The media

Newspapers, books, magazines, television, and radio (for example, Radio 4's *You and Yours*) aim to entertain, inform, and instruct. Although they are passive forms of communication, when used selectively, they may be useful in providing practical information about a wide range of interests and give temporary relief from stress by diverting attention from worries.

Ideas for relieving stress and coping with worries, disabilities, handicaps, and health and family matters are constantly being discussed, and through letters and "talk in" programmes, individual problems can also be dealt with. Notice boards in local libraries are often a good source of information about local helping agencies and facilities.

The telephone

The telephone gives confidential access to an enormous number of helping organisations nationwide. It is particularly useful for overcoming the initial reluctance and embarrassment of seeking outside information and support.

The most notable source of confidential telephone contact is the Samaritans. The organisation has a comprehensive network of contacts with other agencies and the caring professions. Its 24 hour telephone service is provided in the main by part-time volunteers of all ages from all walks of life, who have some training but whose main strength lies in their willingness to listen sympathetically, without imposing their views on the caller.

The family doctor

For many people under stress, particularly those with no or few confidants, the family doctor becomes the first and the chief source of help. Doctors deal with all aspects of life that affect health, but like other people they vary in their reaction to the stress responses they have to treat.

Most prefer to deal with stress by counselling and general advice. Even the act of giving a full account of the circumstances surrounding the stress, with the doctor listening carefully to the descriptions, is usually helpful because it assists us to get the stress in perspective, so that we can begin to adjust and make decisions. It is also reassuring to find out from the doctor that we do not have any serious illness.

The doctor may, in a few cases, arrange for special blood tests or heart checks. To us, the signs of stress may seem overwhelming and certain to mean disease, and it is reassuring to know that nothing serious is amiss and that the body is functioning perfectly efficiently—even under stress. Some doctors may decide not to investigate a patient's general health, judging that the stress is not a sign of underlying disease. It is a matter of clinical judgement, and all our circumstances are different.

False friends

Smoking tobacco, drinking excess alcohol, and taking drugs of dependence (sometimes even those prescribed by the doctor, if not carefully monitored) are unhealthy, unwise, and should be stopped or severely curtailed. They are false friends because they provide the illusion of temporary relief from stress, while in reality making the processes of defence and successful adaptation much more difficult.

People under stress sometimes attempt to cope either deliberately or unconsciously by using these substances to deal with the symptoms they experience or to withstand the pressure they feel under.

Alcohol

Alcohol in moderation may be a pleasure but it is a potentially addictive drug with many subtle and complicated effects. Any long standing stressful situation invites the serious risk of heavy drinking and eventual dependence on alcohol, which may wreck marriages, family and social life, careers, and health (and of course you should never drive after drinking).

A "unit" of alcohol may be defined as the equivalent of half a pint of beer or cider (of normal strength), or a single measure of sherry, Martini, etc, or a single measure of spirits, or a small glass of wine. The average man or woman will react to units of alcohol as shown in the Table, with women affected at lower "doses" than men and the effects being increased by factors such as lack of food, tiredness, and stress.

Units consumed	Effects
1–2	Enhanced sense of wellbeing, but reaction time noticeably reduced.
2–4	Some loss of inhibition with impaired judgement. Accidents become more likely.
3–5	Noticeable loss of inhibition, with physical incoordination. Beyond the legal limit for driving.
4–7	Loss of physical control and clumsiness. Obviously drunk, with extreme reactions. Above this level there is progressive loss of consciousness by degrees.

Dependence on alcohol

The main signs that you may be developing a dependence on alcohol are listed below. Not all these signs may be present and any one may occur to variable degrees in different people.

● Subjective awareness of a compulsion to drink
● Narrowing and stereotyping of the daily drinking pattern or what you drink
● Drinking takes priority over other activities
● Tolerance for alcohol changes—this usually increases at first but eventually falls
● Repeated symptoms of alcohol withdrawal—nausea, headache, nervousness, shaking, sweating, tenseness, jitteriness, being on "edge"
● Relief or avoidance of withdrawal symptoms by further drinking

● Rapid return of the features of dependence after a period of abstinence

"Safe drinking"
Safe levels of drinking are difficult to define precisely for each person and depend on factors such as sex, body size, and constitution. The levels are lower for women than for men.

Approximately one pint of ordinary beer or two single (pub) measures of spirits, or two small glasses of wine per day (ie two units) are reasonable, safe limits. Remember that what others choose to drink is irrelevant to your health and try to find some non-alcoholic alternative for lengthy "drinking" sessions.

A man who drinks eight or more units a day (50 a week) or a woman who drinks more than five a day (35 a week) is at great risk of developing an alcohol related problem.

Cutting down on drinking

1. Keep a diary of your daily drinking—how much, how long, and where.

2. Draw up a time table and:

   a. Reduce the overall amount by stopping drinking at certain times, for example lunch time, and do something else instead;

   b. Limit yourself to a set number of drinks each day—bearing in mind the guidelines for safe drinking—and have at least two alcohol free days each week;

   c. Allow yourself only one alcoholic drink an hour at any drinking occasion;

   d. Avoid drinking in "rounds" if you are likely to break the above rules;

e. Drink a long soft drink to quench your thirst before starting on alcohol;

f. Add mixers to wines and spirits to increase the volume and so help slow down consumption.

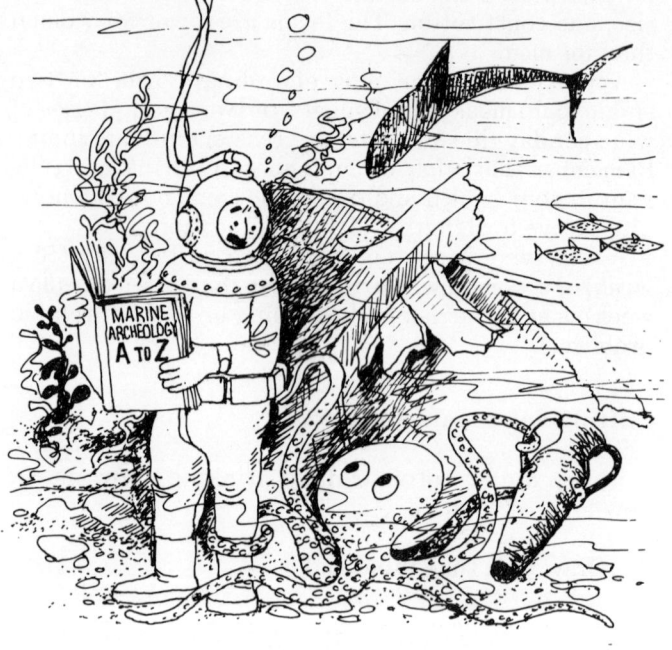

3. Keep busy, plan activities that will keep your mind off drink.

4. Avoid reminders of drinking and whenever possible places where alcohol will be consumed or people who will offer you a drink. Plan avoiding action for times when you are confronted by these situations.

You may find it useful to involve a supportive relative or friend who can put up a united resistance with you.

Tobacco

The most common reason that cigarette smokers give for not stopping smoking is stress, but cutting out (or certainly cutting down) smoking should be the number one health priority. Tell a smoker that his habit is killing him, however, and the first thing he will probably do is light a cigarette.

The most important step in giving up is the decision that you really do want to stop. Unfortunately the reasons for stopping smoking actually make it harder to stop. Firstly because they create a feeling of sacrifice (being forced to give up a little friend, prop, pleasure, or however the smoker views cigarettes) and secondly because they create a blind—we do not smoke for the reasons we should stop—which prevents us from asking ourselves the real reasons for wanting or needing to smoke.

Initially, forget the "sensible" reasons for stopping and ask yourself;

1. What is smoking doing for me?

2. Do I actually enjoy it?

3. Do I really need to go through life spending a fortune just to stick these things in my mouth and make myself ill?

Remember that you had no need to smoke before you became hooked. The first cigarette probably tasted awful and you had to work quite hard to become addicted. The most annoying part is that non-smokers do not seem to be missing out on anything; in fact smokers keep smoking to achieve the same state of "tranquillity" as non-smokers. So why do you smoke? Forget about stress, boredom, and all the other reasons you may think you have, there are two real reasons— nicotine addiction and brainwashing.

Nicotine addiction

Nicotine is one of the fastest acting addictive drugs known to mankind. The concentration in the bloodstream falls quickly, however, to about half some 30 minutes after finishing a cigarette and to only a quarter within an hour.

The withdrawal pangs from nicotine are so subtle that most smokers do not even realise that they are drug addicts. Fortunately it is a relatively easy drug to "kick" once you have accepted that this is the case. There is no physical pain, merely an empty restless feeling, the feeling of something missing. If withdrawal is prolonged the smoker becomes nervous, insecure, agitated, lacking in confidence, and irritable. Within seconds of lighting a cigarette nicotine is supplied resulting in the feeling of relaxation and confidence that the cigarette gives. As soon as this cigarette is put out the chain starts again. The difficulty is that it is when you are not smoking you suffer the feelings and you do not therefore blame the cigarette. When you light up you obtain relief and are fooled into believing that the cigarette is the cure for the bad feelings.

So we smoke to feed the little monster, but we decide when to do it and we do it more during stressful situations, when we need to concentrate, when we are bored, and when we wish to relax.

Brainwashing

Nicotine addiction is not the only problem and it is relatively easy to cope with (the smoker does not, for instance, wake up through the night craving for a cigarette). Another major difficulty is "brainwashing". The subconscious is a very powerful element in our minds and despite anti-smoking campaigns we are still bombarded with extremely clever advertising which tells us that cigarettes relax us and give us confidence, and that the most precious thing on earth is a cigarette. Once addicted to nicotine the power of the advertising is increased, enforcing the fear of giving up.

NO SMOKING

Giving up

1. Decide that you really want to do it and realise that you can achieve your goal. Remember that smokers are not weak willed and that it is only the indecision and moping that make giving up more difficult.

2. Recognise and think about the fact that you are addicted to nicotine but remember that withdrawal is not as painful as you think it is going to be and that it takes only about three weeks to rid the body of 99% of the nicotine.

3. Look forward to the freedom. Do not be afraid of losing the prop you have been brainwashed into believing you need. Smoking enslaves you, preventing you from achieving the peace and confidence you had as a non-smoker.

4. Stop smoking completely. Remember there is no such thing as just one cigarette, smoking is a drug addiction and a chain reaction. By moping about the one cigarette you will be punishing yourself needlessly.

5. Watch out for smokers—they may feel threatened by the fact that you have given up and may try to tempt you back.

6. Keep reminding yourself that there is nothing to give up, on the contrary there are enormous positive gains to be made by not smoking.

Drugs

We are experiencing an increasing national dependence on drugs, pills, and painkillers of all kinds. We are in danger of reaching the point where we believe that every ache, pain, or worry must be soothed away by taking some kind of preparation, encouraging the idea that any form of stress is harmful. There is a strong link between an overtly pill conscious society and one that includes a growing number of drug addicts. Some varieties of sleeping tablets and tranquillisers (such as *valium* and *librium*) show this connection by the pleasurable effects they induce in vulnerable people. Experiencing these effects may lead to dependence and can bring all the complications of dependence on stronger drugs, including withdrawal symptoms if they are stopped and a desperate need to have a good supply in case they are needed.

Occasionally a mild tranquilliser, sleeping pills, or antidepressants may be prescribed by the family doctor to relieve the symptoms of stress. This will almost always be because the stress response has been established and the "cycle" needs to be interrupted, usually only for a short period. These are temporary remedies for stress and in the absence of clear cut medical conditions cannot be assumed to cure stress—especially when there are outside physical, emotional, and social factors operating. Drugs may be helpful in tiding people over a crisis and allowing them some rest and respite from overwhelming feelings of stress. In these circumstances the drugs are more likely to be beneficial than harmful. Generally, however, doctors and patients have become more aware of the problem of dependency and so less of these drugs are being prescribed. This is in line with the general opinion that self-help methods are both more appropriate and safer for coping with stress.

Some golden rules for reducing stress

Get your priorities right—sort out what really matters in your life

Think ahead and try to anticipate how to get round difficulties

Share your worries with family or friends whenever possible

Stay sober, "drowning your sorrows" will not help you

Seek information, help and advice early, even though it takes an effort

Try to develop a social network or circle of friends

Take up hobbies and interests

Exercise regularly

Eat good, wholesome food

Lead a regular life-style

Give yourself treats and rewards for positive actions, attitudes, and thoughts

Don't regard difficulties as personal failings or failures—they are challenges to improve your ingenuity and stamina

Don't be too hard on yourself—try to keep things in proportion

Get to know yourself better—improve your defences and strengthen your weak points

Don't "bottle things up" or sit all night brooding—think realistically about problems and decide to take some appropriate action; if necessary distract yourself in some pleasant way

Don't be reluctant to seek medical help if you are worried about your health

Remember that there are many people who have faced similar circumstances and have dealt with them successfully, with or without the help of others

There are always people who are willing and able to help whatever the problem—don't be unwilling to benefit from their experience

Conclusion

Although we cannot, and indeed must not, avoid stress we can learn to meet it efficiently and live with it successfully rather than letting stress overwhelm us to the extent that it affects our mental and physical health adversely. Some useful rules for avoiding or reducing stress are set out on the previous page.

Because of the enormous individual differences in what causes us stress and in our ability to cope, this booklet cannot hope to give the answer to everyone's problems. What it has tried to do, however, is to help the reader think about and identify the undesirable stresses in his or her own life and learn how to control these—either alone or with the help of others. Taking stock of ourselves and our lives from time to time can be an extremely beneficial exercise. It is amazing how little we question our priorities and how many sources of unnecessary stress we can be rid of by doing this.

Other booklets available in the Family Doctor series:

Understanding rheumatism

Life with asthma

Heart attack—prevention and treatment

Depression and its treatment

Knowing about sex

Teenage living and loving

Contraception choice not chance

Women only

Looking at retirement

Life with diabetes

Children's disorders of the throat and ear

You and your bowels

AIDS

The facts about drugs

Arthritis and joint replacement

You and your blood pressure

Migraine and other headaches

Infertility and in vitro fertilisation

Available from chemists or direct from:

Family Doctor Publications, BMA House, Tavistock Square, London WC1H 9JP.